LEARNING GENERAL PRACTICE

A Structured Approach for Trainee GPs and Trainers

LEARNING GENERAL PRACTICE

A Structured Approach for Trainee GPs and Trainers

JOHN SANDARS MB ChB(Hons) MRCP(UK) MRCGP
Trainer in General Practice
Cheadle Hulme Health Centre, Stockport, Cheshire.
Clinical Tutor in General Practice, Stockport, Cheshire.
Chairman, Education Subcommittee, North West
Faculty of the Royal College of General Practitioners.

REBECCA BARON MB ChB DRCOG MRCGP
General Practitioner, Stockport, Cheshire.
Previously Trainee in General Practice,
Cheadle Hulme Health Centre, Stockport, Cheshire.

PASTEST SERVICE

© 1988 PASTEST SERVICE
304 Galley Hill
Hemel Hempstead, Hertfordshire
Telephone: 0442-52113

First published 1988

British Library Cataloguing in Publication Data
Sandars, John
Learning general practice.
1. Medicine. Questions & answers - for general practice
I. Title II. Baron, Rebecca
610'.76

ISBN 0-906896-41-X

Text prepared by Turner Associates, Knutsford, Cheshire.
Printed by Martins, Berwick upon Tweed.

Contents

TUTORIAL CHECKLIST: Please tick each box as you complete a tutorial.

Introduction

In order to maximise the learning opportunities of the Trainee year in General Practice it is essential that the Trainee covers the wide field of General Practice in a methodical way.

This book of tutorials has been designed to help Trainers and Trainees alike to adopt a systematic approach to covering all the necessary information that a Trainee could be expected to know by the end of the year.

Each Tutorial has a common format:

> Learning Objectives: These are the key aspects of knowledge that the Trainee should be expected to know.
>
> Skills Required: The Trainee should be expected to have acquired these skills by the end of the trainee year.
>
> Trainee Self Awareness: These questions are designed to prompt discussions of key areas e.g. by considering clinical problems in their physical, psychological and social terms, and by appreciating the moral and ethical dimensions which affect their decisions.
>
> Further Reading: The titles chosen have particular relevance to General Practice and are comprehensive enough to provide basic knowledge relevant to the MRCGP examination.

It is suggested that the Trainer and Trainee together choose a Tutorial for discussion at their next meeting. The chosen Tutorial should be prepared by the Trainee prior to the meeting by reading the titles in the Further Reading section and then checking in the Tutorial that the key Learning Objectives and Skills have been acquired, together with an understanding of the subject as detailed in Trainee Self Awareness.

Each Tutorial contains brief notes and pointers to indicate to the Trainee the basic knowledge required on any given topic, whether it be clinical or practice management related.

The points listed will provide the Trainee with a framework on which to build up his or her knowledge. Each point should initiate further investigation in order for the Trainee to learn the basic knowledge required for a comprehensive understanding of the chosen topic.

Only when the essential groundwork has been covered can the Trainer and Trainee maximise the potential of each tutorial. By using the Tutorial checklist, the trainee can keep track of his progress and produce an individual syllabus for learning.

Assessment of the Trainee is becoming increasingly important; the Checklist and 60 Multiple Choice Question Paper can provide an initial, and a later assessment.

We hope this book will provide both trainers and trainees with a stimulating tool to learn general practice and we would like to thank Dr John Day, Course Organiser Stockport Vocational Training Scheme for his helpful comments and criticism.

The Nature of General Practice

Definition of the General Practitioner:

"The general practitioner is a licensed medical graduate who gives personal, primary and continuing care to individuals, families and a practice population, irrespective of age, sex and illness. It is the synthesis of these functions which is unique. He will attend his patients in his consulting room and in their home and sometimes in a clinic or a hospital. His aim is to make early diagnoses. He will include and integrate physical, psychological and social factors in his considerations about health and illness. This will be expressed in the care of his patients. He will make an initial decision about every problem which is presented to him as a doctor. He will undertake the continuing management of his patients with chronic, recurrent or terminal illness. Prolonged contact means that he can use repeated opportunities to gather information at a pace appropriate to each patient and build up a relationship of trust which he can use professionally. He will practice in cooperation with other colleagues, medical and non medical. He will know how and when to intervene through treatment, prevention and education to promote the health of his patients and their families. He will recognise that he also has a professional responsibility to the community".

The educational needs of the future general practitioner. Journal of the Royal College of General Practitioners 18, 358 (1969). Reproduced with permission from the Editor.

What is seen in General Practice.

Major illness in a practice of 2500

Conditions		Persons consulting per year
Acute Bronchitis		100
Pneumonia		20
Severe Depression		10
Suicide attempt		3
Suicide 1 every 4 years		
Acute Myocardial Infarction		8
Acute Appendicitis		5
Acute Strokes		5
All new cancers		5
Lung	2 per year	
Breast	1 per year	
Large Bowel	2 every 3 years	
Stomach	1 every 2 years	
Prostate	1 every 2 years	
Bladder	1 every 3 years	
Cervix	1 every 4 years	
Ovary	1 every 5 years	
Oesophagus	1 every 7 years	
Brain	1 every 10 years	
Uterine body	1 every 12 years	
Lymphadenoma	1 every 15 years	
Thyroid	1 every 20 years	

Minor illness in a practice of 2500

Conditions	Persons consulting per year
General	
Upper respiratory infections	600
Skin disorders	325
Emotional disorders	300
Gastro-intestinal disorders	200
Specific	
Acute tonsillitis	100
Acute otitis media	75
Cerumen	50
Acute urinary infections	50
'Acute back' syndrome	50
Migraine	25
Hay fever	25

Chronic disease in a practice of 2500

Conditions	Persons consulting per year
Chronic rheumatism	100
Rheumatoid arthritis	10
Osteoarthritis of hips	5
Chronic mental illness	60
High blood pressure	50
Obesity	40
Chronic bronchitis	35
Anaemia	
Iron deficiency	25
Pernicious anaemia	4
Chronic heart failure	30
Cancers	30
Asthma	25
Peptic ulcers	20
Coronary artery disease	20
Cerebrovascular disease	15
Epilepsy	10
Diabetes	10
Thyroid disease	7
Parkinsonism	3
Multiple sclerosis	2
Chronic renal failure	less than 1

The 3 tables above have been reproduced with permission from 'A Workbook for Trainees in General Practice' by P. Freeling, published by John Wright.

Further Reading

Common Diseases: their Nature, Incidence and Care. J. Fry. MTP Press.

Present State and Future Needs in General Practice. J. Fry. for RCGP by MTP Press. RCGP Publications.

Tutorial 1: Starting in Practice

Learning Objectives

1. **Finance**
   Tax forms to Practice Manager
   Copy GMC certificate and valid Defence Society certificate

2. **Contract**
   Study leave
   Car expenses
   Telephone expenses

3. **Education**
   Trainer/trainee tutorials
   Postgraduate centre/library
   Day release course
   Special courses
   Attachments: e.g. eye clinic
   JCC (Joint Committee on Contraception). Make arrangements for theoretical and practical training

4. **Practice**
   Structure
   Personnel: Secretarial
   Reception
   Nursing
   Health Visitor
   Midwife
   Meetings
   On call arrangements
   Rotas
   Stationery
   Keys
   Telephone numbers
   Admissions procedures to local hospitals

5. **Dealing with emergencies in practice**
   Advice over telephone
   Management Plans for common emergencies
   Criteria for admission

Further Reading

A Guide to General Practice. Oxford GP Group. Blackwell Scientific.
Emergencies in General Practice. A. J. Moulds, P. B. Martin and T. A. Bouchier-Hayes. MTP Press.

Starting Checklist

Telephone Nos:

(A) **Practice**

Practice Address

Partners

Staff

Family Practitioner Committee

(B) **Local Services**
District Nurse

Midwife

Health Visitor

Police

Ambulance

Telephone Nos:

Social Services ________ Daytime ________

Out of Hours ________

Council for Voluntary Social Service(CVS) ________

Physiotherapists ________

Citizens' Advice Bureau ________

Pharmacists ________

Undertakers ________

Optician ________

Chiropodist ________

Samaritans ________

Marriage Guidance (Relate) ________

Hospitals

____

____

____

____

____

Miscellaneous

____

____

____

____

____

____

Doctor's Bag Checklist

1. Essentials

Stethoscope
Ophthalmoscope/Auriscope
Sphygmomanometer
Torch
Tongue depressors
Disposable gloves
Stationery (practice note paper and envelopes)
Prescription Pad
List of useful telephone numbers
Copy of MIMS/BNF
Temporary Resident forms and Emergency Treatment forms

2. Optional

Thermometer including low reading
Reflex hammer
Urine testing equipment - Clinistix
Blood collecting equipment

3. Emergency Bag

Contents: Individual preference

Further Reading
A Guide to General Practice. Oxford GP Group (1987). Blackwell Scientific.

Your Notes and Questions

Tutorial 2: The Organisation of General Practice

Learning Objectives

1. **Structure, Function and Responsibility**
   Secretary of State for Social Services
   General Medical Council (GMC)
   Family Practitioner Committee (FPC)
   Medical Practices Committee: Restricted/intermediate/open/designated areas
   Community Health Councils (CHC)
   Local Medical Committee (LMC)
   General Medical Services Committee (GMSC)
   Regional Health Authority (RHA)
   District Health Authority (DHA)
   District Management Team
   The Review Body
   British Medical Association (BMA)
   Royal College of General Practitioners (RCGP)

2. **Terms of Service**
   The NHS (General Medical and Pharmaceutical) Regulations 1974
   'The GP Contract'. Available from FPC.

3. **The Patient's View**

Trainee Self Awareness

1. Should every patient requesting a home visit be visited? What are your obligations?
2. For which certificates can a charge be made?
3. Through what channels can a patient make a complaint against a doctor?
4. What is the role of the Community Health Council (CHC)?
5. How can the views of the individual GP be represented to the Government?

Further Reading

SFA (Statement of Fees and Allowances, The Red Book.) Family Practitioner Committee.
Running a Practice. R. V. H. Jones et al. Croom Helm.

Your Notes and Questions

Tutorial 3: Social Services

Learning Objectives

1. **Local Authority Departments**

Director of Social Services via Area Teams
Social Workers Case work concept
Assessment of needs
Responsibilities

1. Work with Children and Families
   Voluntary fostering/ adoption
   Statutory: child committed to care of Local Authority by Courts
   Place of Safety Order if in physical or moral danger or delinquent child

2. Work with Elderly
   Residential. (Part III Accommodation) Elderly Persons Home (EPH)

3. Work with Physically Handicapped
   Blind (see Tutorial 19: Eyes)

4. Work with Mentally Handicapped
   Essential role in Mental Health Act 1983

5. Care of Homeless and Single Parent Families

6. Resources
   Aids and adaptations
   Sheltered housing
   Residential
   Hostels
   Sheltered workshops
   Home Helps
   Meals on Wheels
   Day Centres and Day Nurseries
   Transport including Orange badge
   Dirty Linen Service

2. **Voluntary**

National: NSPCC, WRVS
Local: Coordination by local CVS (Council for Voluntary Service)
CAB (Citizens' Advice Bureau)
Charities and funds

3. **Support of Carers**

A carer is someone whose life is restricted because of the need to look after mentally, physically handicapped or elderly persons.

4. **DHSS (Department of Health and Social Security)**
   Numerous benefits and allowances. Complex rules.
   Main groups:
   - Income supplement
   - Help with Rent and Rates
   - Children/Maternity
   - Illness
   - Lone Parents
   - Injured at work
   - Handicapped or disabled
   - Retirement
   - Widows

Trainee Self Awareness

1. How would you assess the needs of a 'battered wife'? What help could you obtain for her and from where?
2. How would you proceed to get a child taken into care?
3. What is a 'Problem Family' and what help is available to them?

Further Reading
Social Services. A. Byrne and C. Padfield. Made Simple Books: Heinemann.

Your Notes and Questions

Tutorial 4: Forms

Learning Objectives

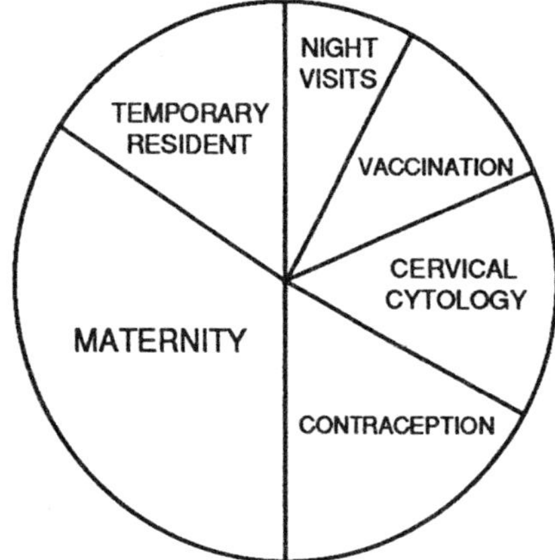

1. Concept of Items of Service
10% of gross annual income

2. Knowledge for Each Item of Service
1. Form for claim
2. Conditions of claim: usually indicated in the Red Book (SFA)
3. Payment for form
   Forms are also detailed in each relevant Tutorial

3. Knowledge of Certification for Incapacity to Work
Outlined in 'Medical Evidence for Social Security Purposes' from DHSS

4. Knowledge of Prescribing
1. How to write a prescription
2. What may or may not be prescribed
   Concept of Limited List
   Concept of ACBS (Advisory Committee on Borderline Substances)
3. What quantities may be prescribed
4. Who is exempted from prescription charges
5. What charges may the patient be required to pay
6. When should a private prescription be issued
7. How may surgical appliances be prescribed see Drug Tariff

Trainee Self Awareness

1. How would you deal with a patient who is requesting a further sick note although you feel that he is 'swinging the lead'?
2. Does maximising income, by increasing item of service fees, lead to better patient care?
3. Do you feel embarrassed when asking patients for fees? Discuss your response.
4. What are the methods of remuneration for dispensing doctors?

Further Reading

SFA (The Red Book). Family Practitioner Committee.
Drug Tariff. DHSS. From Family Practitioner Committee.
'Medical Evidence for Social Security Purposes'. DHSS.
Pulse 'Blue Book': Published yearly by Pulse Magazine.

Your Notes and Questions

Forms Check List

(It is helpful to collect one of each of these forms for familiarisation. Tick off each box as you obtain the relevant form.)

1. Prescriptions

- ☐ FP 10
- ☐ FP 95 — pre-payment application
- ☐ FP 91 — exemptions and refunds
- ☐ FP 57 — receipt for prescription charges

2. Off Work

- ☐ SC 1 — self certification
- ☐ Form Med 3
- ☐ Form Med 5
- ☐ RM 7 — special referrals to Regional Medical Officer
- ☐ Private Sick Notes
- ☐ Special Notes e.g. insurance

3. Maternity SFA 31

- ☐ FW 8 — pregnancy exemption of prescription charges and welfare foods
- ☐ Mat B1 and 2 — expected confinement/confinement
- ☐ FP 24 — on obstetric list
- ☐ FP 24A — not on obstetric list

4. Administrative

- ☐ FP 1 — acceptance form
- ☐ FP 5 and 6 — medical record envelope (Men and Women)
- ☐ FP 7 and 8 — continuation card (Men and Women)
- ☐ FP 7A and 8A — summary of immunisation card (Men and Women)
- ☐ FP 9A and 9B — summary of treatment card (Men and Women)
- ☐ FP 30 — requisition for forms
- ☐ FP 34 — invoice relating to drugs (dispensing)
- ☐ FP 34D — invoice relating to drugs (non-dispensing) SFA 44

5. Contraception

- ☐ FP 1001 — ordinary
- ☐ FP 1001 — IUCD SFA 29
- ☐ FP 1003 — treatment of temporary resident

6. Immunisation

- ☐ FP 73 SFA 27
- ☐ International Certificate of Vaccination against Cholera

7. Other Forms for which Fee Claimable

- ☐ FP 81 — night visit SFA 24
- ☐ FP 32 — emergency treatment SFA 33
- ☐ FP 19 — temporary resident SFA 32
- ☐ FP 74 — cervical cytology SFA 28
- ☐ DTp 200002 — exemption to wear seat belt
- ☐ Cremation Certificate: Part 1 and Part 2
- ☐ BUPA/PPP claim forms

8. Other Forms for which no fee is claimable

- ☐ Death Certificate
- ☐ Certificate A Abortion Act 1967 (HSA 1)
- ☐ Recommendation: supply of invalid vehicle
- ☐ Applications for Special Grants from DHSS

9. Pathology/X-Ray/Physiotherapy Request Forms

Your Notes and Questions

Tutorial 5: Practice Administration

Learning Objectives

1. **Medical Records**
   - Filing systems
   - Organisation
   - Medical record envelope FP 5 and 6
   - A4 Records
   - Computers
   - Structured records
   - Summary cards
   - Feature cards e.g. Planned care for Hypertension
   - Diagnostic Index
   - Age-sex Index
   - Disease Register

2. **Use of Computers**

3. **Appointment Systems**

4. **Home Visits**
   - Out of Hours
   - Re-visit
   - Regular/Routine Visiting

5. **Repeat Prescriptions**
   - Common drugs
     - acting on CNS
     - antihypertensives
     - antirheumatics
   - Drug cards
   - Drug registers
   - Concept of Balint 'Treatment or Diagnosis'. Patient never comes to doctor but continues to ask for repeat prescriptions
     - (a) hostile doctor/patient relationship
     - (b) patient and doctor make implicit 'contract' not to discuss previous medical (often psychosocial) problems or offer new problems

6. **Deputising Services**

7. **Staff**

Trainee Self Awareness

1. How would you deal with staff complaints?
2. What are the likely explanations of a sudden dramatic increase in night visits? How would you determine the cause?
3. What are the advantages and disadvantages, to doctor and patient, of deputising services?

4. To what extent can home visits be delegated?
5. How may bad medical records result in bad medical care?

Further Reading

Practice Management. P. Pritchard. Oxford University Press.
Organising a Practice. BMJ Publications.
Running a Practice. R. V. H. Jones et al. Croom Helm.
The Use of Computers in General Practice (1983). J Preece. (Library of General Practice, vol. 5) Churchill Livingstone.
Treatment or Diagnosis. M. Balint et al. Tavistock Publications.
RCGP Information Folders : Age/Sex Registers
Appointment Systems
Medical Records
Practice Information Booklets.

Your Notes and Questions

Tutorial 6: The Finances of General Practice

Learning Objectives

1. Income

- FPC Income
  - Capitation fees
  - Basic and special allowances
    - Basic practice allowance
    - Group practice allowance
    - Seniority/postgraduate/vocational allowance
    - Supplementary practice allowance
    - Designated area allowance
  - Items of service fees (see Tutorial 4: Forms)
  - Others
    - Leave payment
    - Rural practice payments
    - Dispensing income
- Work Outside Practice
  - Hospital work e.g. clinical assistant
  - Government work e.g. medical board
  - Private e.g. life insurance
    - PSV/HGV
    - Cremations
    - Legal reports
- Reimbursement of GP Expenses
  - Staff costs
  - Cost of premises
    - Health centres
    - Cost rent
    - Notional rent

2. Expenses

- Staff
- Premises
- Services e.g. telephone
- Professional e.g. societies, drugs and dressings
- Capital expenses

3. Taxation

4. Practice Accounts

5. Premises

- Improvement of surgery premises
- Cost rent scheme

Skills

Ability to read Profit and Loss account of practice.

Trainee Self Awareness

1. What are the advantages and disadvantages of Health Authority owned health centres compared with privately owned premises?
2. How can the building of privately owned premises be financed?
3. What is meant by the term 'independent contractor' and what are its implications?
4. Many GPs are said to receive less income than they are entitled to? How might this arise? How can you ensure that this does not happen in your practice?

Further Reading
SFA (The Red Book). Family Practitioner Committee.
Running a Practice. R. V. H. Jones et al. Croom Helm.

Your Notes and Questions

Tutorial 7: The Primary Care Team

Learning Objectives

A definition of the Primary Care Team:

"The practice team consists of a core of individuals in different professions each working from a base in the same building. In addition there are other colleagues who come to the practice building to see the patients of that practice. The core team usually consists of general practitioners, practice nurses, community nurses and health visitors with practice administrators/managers and secretarial and reception staff. In some practices midwives, counsellors and psychiatric nurses may be members of the core team."
Para 5.2 Reports from General Practice 25. RCGP Publication.

1. **Knowledge of Training and Roles**
   District (Community) Nurses
   Bath Nurses
   Practice Nurses
   Midwives
   Health Visitors
   Community Psychiatric Nurses (CPN)
   Practice Administrator/Manager
   Medical Secretaries
   Receptionists

2. **The GP as an Employer**
   The type of staff employed
   Recruitment
   Training
   Contracts
   Pay
   Management heirarchy

3. **The principles of management in practice**

Trainee Self Awareness

1. What duties do you think the practice nurse should undertake in the treatment room?
2. How many ancillary staff should be employed in a practice and what are the regulations regarding their remuneration?
3. What are your legal obligations as an employer?
4. What is AMSPAR? How may it help your staff?
5. You decide that you need to employ a new receptionist. How would you go about filling this vacancy?

Further Reading
Employing Staff. N. Ellis. BMJ Publications.

Running a Practice. R. V. H. Jones et al. Croom Helm.
Management in Practice. RCGP Video Package 1987. (Discusses the dynamics and difficulties of setting up a Diabetic Mini-Clinic.)

Your Notes and Questions

Tutorial 8: Medico-Legal Aspects

Learning Objectives

1. **Certification**
   Incapacity Certificates: private and statutory
   Death Certificate
   Cremation Certificate
   Role of Coroner

2. **Writing Legal Reports**

3. **Principles of Confidentiality**

4. **Principles of Consent**

5. **Contracts**
   Patients and NHS via FPC
   Partners
   Employed staff
   Trainee

6. **Prescribing**
   Misuse of Drugs Act

Trainee Self Awareness

1. Should patients have the right to see their own notes?
2. A 22 year old nurse asks you to remove all mention of her recent abortion from your records. How would you respond?
3. What are your legal obligations when treating a drug addict?
4. What are the different types of consent and when is the use of each appropriate?

Further Reading

Running a Practice. R. V. H. Jones et al. Croom Helm.
Professional Conduct and Discipline: fitness to practice: GMC.
The Handbook of Medical Ethics. BMJ Publications.
Medical Aspects of Fitness to Drive. Medical Commission on Accident Prevention.
Lecture Notes on Forensic Medicine. D. Gee. Blackwell Scientific Publications.

Your Notes and Questions

Tutorial 9: Psycho-social Crisis Intervention

Learning Objectives

1. Crisis = upset in steady state by a stressor:

e.g. a) during life cycle transitions, e.g. marriage
b) loss, e.g. death, illness, self esteem
c) family conflict

2. Model of a Crisis

Impact
Disorganisation
disbelief
anger/agitation
confusion
Recovery
either resolves as a challenge and leads to personal growth
or leads to mental illness

3. Management Plan

Be prepared and allow adequate time
Show concern and allow ventilation of feelings
Remain calm
Assess whether there is a true emergency
medical emergency?
suicidal or psychiatric emergency?
consider urgent admission? Mental Health Act (MHA) section?
Encourage specificity of problems

Jointly agree on practical solutions to problems, make appropriate referral, e.g. Social Workers, Citizens Advice Bureau.

Offer continuing support:
self - including consideration of medication
support network - e.g. Samaritans, local Church

When out of hours try to avoid making a crisis out of a problem which is really a long term one.

Trainee Self Awareness

1. You are called out to see a 90 year old lady who has just been burgled. How would you assess the situation and how might you manage it?
2. What do you know about the Samaritans?
3. How might you contact Social Services out of hours and what help would you expect them to be able to offer?

Further Reading
Organisations and Self Help Groups, see Appendix 2.

Tutorial 10: The Consultation

Learning Objectives

Theoretical models help us to understand and analyse what is happening when a patient consults a doctor.

1. **Description of events occurring in a consultation** (after Byrne and Long):

   The doctor establishes a relationship with the patient.

   The doctor either attempts to discover, or actually discovers, the reason for the patient's attendance.

   The doctor conducts a verbal, or physical examination, or both.

   The doctor, or the doctor and the patient, or the patient (usually in that order of probability) consider(s) the condition.

   The doctor, and occasionally the patient, details treatment or further investigation.

   The consultation is terminated, usually by the doctor.

2. **Expansion to include Preventative Medicine** (after Stott and Davis):
   Management of presenting problems
   Management of continuing problems
   Modification of help-seeking behaviour
   Opportunistic health promotion

3. **A model of seven tasks** to be completed for an effective consultation, based on the patient's health understanding (after Pendleton).
   To define the reasons for the patient's attendance, including:
      the nature and history of the problem
      their cause
      the patient's ideas, concerns and expectations
      the effects of the problems.
   To consider other problems:
      continuing problems
      'at risk' factors.
   To choose with the patient an appropriate action for each problem.
   To achieve a shared understanding of the problem with the patient.
   To involve the patient in the management plan and encourage him to accept appropriate responsibility.
   To use time and resources appropriately.
   To establish or maintain a relationship with the patient which helps to achieve the other tasks.

4. **Transactional Analysis,** helping to understand why communication may break down (after Berne)

5. **Balint.** Based on the recognition and acceptance of feelings, both of the patient and the doctor, in the consultation. (see Tutorial 11.)

Skills

Awareness of what is happening, both in the nature of a problem and why the patient brings a problem. Also how you feel about the patient and how this affects your subsequent consultation.

Use of audio and/or video taping of consultations.

Trainee Self Awareness

1. Do you find yourself becoming angry if the patient thinks he has a physical problem and he hasn't? Why do you feel the way you do?
2. Can there be more than one 'patient' presented to you? How do you manage this situation?
3. Discuss 'if you ask questions all you get is answers'
4. Think of a consultation that you felt went well and also one that you felt went badly. Using the above models, why was there a difference?
5. Tape (either audio or video) a random consultation and then analyse it, using the given models.
6. During your next surgery keep a log, e.g.

Name	Symptoms	Actual reason for coming	Why now
F. Smith	Headache	Worried re impotence	Wife just left him

Further Reading

Games People Play. E. Berne. Penguin.
The Consultation. D. Pendleton et al. Oxford University Press.
Doctors talking to patients. P. S. Byrne and B. E. L. Long. RCGP ublications.
The Exceptional Potential in Each Primary Care Consultation. N. C. H. Stott and R. H. Davies. Journal of the RCGP 29:201-5 (1979).
Doctor-Patient Relationship. P. Freeling and M. Harris. Churchill Livingstone.
The Doctor, the Patient and the Illness. M. Balint. Pitman. (see Tutorial 11)
The Inner Consultation. R. Neighbour. MTP Press

Your Notes and Questions

Tutorial 11: Balint

Learning Objectives

Knowledge of Concepts:

1. **"The Doctor as the Drug".** 'Pharmacology' through the Doctor-Patient relationship.

2. **"The Child as the Presenting Complaint".** The patient may offer another person as the problem when there are underlying psycho-social problems.

3. **"Elimination by Appropriate Physical Examination".** This may reinforce the patient's belief that his symptoms (neurotic in origin) are in fact due to physical illness. Repeated investigations perpetuate this cycle.

4. **"Collusion of Anonymity".** As above, referral reinforces mistaken belief in the origin of symptoms. The responsibility of uncovering underlying psycho-social problems becomes increasingly diluted by repeated referral, with nobody taking final responsibility.

5. **"The Mutual Investment Company".** This is formed and managed by the doctor and the patient. "Clinical illnesses" are episodes in a long relationship, and represent "offers" of problems (physical and psycho-social) to the doctor.

6. **"The Flash".** The point in the consultation when the real reason of the "offer" (underlying Psycho-social and neurotic illness) is suddenly apparent to both doctor and patient. This forms a fulcrum for change; the consultation can now deal with the underlying basic "fault".

Skills

General Practice Psychotherapy

- "The Doctor as the Drug"
- Use of a psychological language that the patient understands
- Role of advice and reassurance
- Skill of listening "He who asks questions will only get answers"
- Offer of a long interview. This will be time effective in the long term.
- When to stop
- When to ask for help: Balint group
Psychiatrist

Trainee Self Awareness

1. Assess a recent surgery for possible neurotic symptoms behind the "offer" of physical illness.
2. Review your last "problem case" referral. Was this diluting your responsibility?
3. When did you last experience a "flash" in a consultation? What use did you and the patient make of it?

Further Reading
The Doctor, his Patient and the Illness. M. Balint. Pitman.
Six Minutes for the Patient: Interactions in General Practice Consultation. E. Balint. Tavistock Publications.

Your Notes and Questions

Tutorial 12: GP Psychiatry

Learning Objectives

1. **Knowledge of Natural History**
   - Anxiety
   - Depression
   - Schizophrenia
   - Dementia
   - Post-natal depression

2. **Knowledge of Therapeutics**
   - Tranquillizers
   - Antidepressants
   - Long term (often shared care)
     1. Lithium
     2. Depot Major Tranquillizers

3. **Mental Health Team concept.**
   Role and method of referral:
   - Practice Counsellor
   - Community Psychiatric Nurse (CPN)
   - Clinical Psychologist
   - Social Worker
   - Consultant Psychiatrist

4. **Management Plans**
   - Anxiety
   - Depression
   - Dementia
   - Mental handicap

5. **Indications for referral to Consultant Psychiatrist**

6. **Acute psychiatric emergencies,** especially out of hours
   - Violent/aggressive patients
   - Suicidal: assessment of risk

7. **Use of Mental Health Act 1983**
   - Knowledge of sections: indications
     procedures
   - Role of the social worker

Skills

Basic counselling skills

Trainee Self Awareness

1. What are your indications for prescribing benzodiazepines? How can you monitor your

prescribing? How do you deal with patients with long term use?
2. What is meant by suicide and parasuicide? How can you assess the risk?
3. When would you consider compulsory admission to a mental hospital? How would you arrange this?
4. What is the role of self-help groups for patients with chronic anxiety? How can your patient contact a local group?

Further Reading

Textbook of Psychiatry. M. Gelder et al. Oxford University Press.
Counselling: A Skills Approach. E. Munro et al. Methuen.
The Presentation of Depression: Current Approaches. Occasional Paper 36. RCGP Publications.
The Work of Counsellors in General Practice. Occasional Paper 37. RCGP Publications.

Your Notes and Questions

Tutorial 13: Alcohol and Drug Addiction

Learning Objectives

1. **Knowledge of Risk Factors**
   Physical, Psychological, Social

2. **Problems of Early Identification**
   Use of CAGE questionnaire

3. **Concept of safe drinking limits**

4. **Problem Drinking versus Alcohol Addiction**

5. **Presentation and effects**
   Physical, Psychological, Social, Legal

6. **Management Plans**
   1. General Practitioner
   2. Local services:
      Community Psychiatric Nurse
      Consultant Psychiatrist
      District Team and Centre
   3. Self Help: AA (Alcoholics Anonymous)
   4. Support for Relatives: Al-Anon
   5. Voluntary: Hostels
   6. Legal Aspects
      'Drink Driving'
      Misuse of Drugs Act
      Notification of Addicts
   7. Local method of referral

Skills

Writing out DDA prescriptions

Trainee Self Awareness

1. How can you ask a patient about their alcohol history without putting them on the defensive?
2. What are the advantages and disadvantages of referring alcohol and drug addicts to specialist services, rather than to their own general practitioner?
3. It is often the patient's relatives who first bring the problem to your attention. What difficulties does this create for you, and how do you cope with this?
4. How do you deal with the drug addict who threatens you with violence?
5. A patient attends evening surgery smelling strongly of alcohol and holding a set of car keys. What do you do?

Further Reading

ABC of Alcohol. BMJ Publications.
Alcohol, a balanced view (1986): Reports from General Practice 24. RCGP Publications.
Drug Addiction and Polydrug Abuse. The Role of the GP. A. Banks and T. A. N. Waller. Institute for the Study of Drug Dependency.

Alcoholics Anonymous, see Appendix 2.
Al-Anon, see Appendix 2.

Your Notes and Questions

Tutorial 14: Minor Illness in General Practice

Learning Objectives

1. **Natural History and Management Plans**
   Dizziness
   Diarrhoea and vomiting
   Migraine
   "Tired all the time"
   Threadworms
   Aphthous ulcers

2. **Common Minor Paediatric Problems**
   Temper tantrums
   Sleep problems
   Minor orthopaedic problems

3. **Concept of presentation due to underlying psycho-social problems**

4. **Symptom presentation in General Practice**
   "Tip of the Iceberg"
   Health Belief Model

Trainee Self Awareness

1. What are the common causes of a patient complaining of being "tired all the time?" How would you try to find an underlying cause?
2. What is the place of sedatives in children with sleeping problems?

Further Reading

Practice, A Handbook of Primary Medical Care. J. Cormack et al. Kluwer Medical.
Commonsense Paediatrics. M. Pollak and J. Fry. MTP Press.
Common Diseases: their nature, incidence and care. J. Fry. MTP Press.

Your Notes and Questions

Tutorial 15: Skin diseases

Learning Objectives

1. **Natural History and Management Plans**
   - Acne
   - Eczema
   - Infections, infestations and fungal
   - Psoriasis
   - Leg ulcers
   - Warts and veruccas
   - Pigmented lesions and skin malignancy
   - Herpes-simplex and zoster
   - Skin markers of internal disease
   - Urticaria
   - Napkin rash

2. **Referral**
   - What
   - When
   - To whom: e.g. dermatologist or plastic surgeon

3. **Principles of Therapeutics**

4. **Role of Self Help Groups:**
   - Psoriasis Association
   - Eczema Association

Skills

Skin scrapings and microscopy
Minor operations:
- excision
- cautery
- curettage
- ingrowing toenails

Trainee Self Awareness

1. "Can I have some more Betnovate for that rash on my face?" How do you respond?
2. What are your criteria for referring pigmented lesions to hospital?
3. Can dietary restriction be helpful in the management of skin diseases?
4. What dermatological preparations can be bought over the counter at the local chemist? When would you recommend this rather than give a prescription?
5. Does your treatment plan for mild acne in a 16 year old school boy differ from that in a 22 year old fashion model? What factors influence your treatment?

Further Reading

Practical Dermatology. I. Sneddon and R. Church. Edward Arnold.
Atlas of Dermatology. G. M. Levene and C. D. Calnan. Wolff.
Clinical Dermatology: An Illustrated Textbook. R. McKie. Oxford University Press.

Tutorial 16: Infectious diseases

Learning Objectives

1. **Knowledge of Natural History, Epidemiology and General Practice Management**

   Childhood Exanthems:
   - Rubella
   - Chickenpox
   - Measles
   - Mumps
   - Hepatitis
   - Herpes Simplex
   - Herpes Zoster
   - Whooping Cough
   - Glandular Fever
   - Influenza
   - Hand, Foot and Mouth Disease

2. **Indications for referral**

   Acute admissions of the ill patient

3. **Statutory Notification of Infectious Diseases to Community Physician**

4. **Incubation and Infectivity periods**

5. **Knowledge of common tropical diseases seen in the UK**

6. **Knowledge of 'post-viral syndrome'**

Trainee Self Awareness

1. A patient has just returned from Indonesia and has a high temperature and headache. How would you manage this problem?
2. What are the therapeutic options available to a patient with recurrent herpes simplex around the mouth? Which would you favour and why?
3. What is your management of 'Monospot' negative glandular fever?

Further Reading

Infectious Diseases in General Practice. D. Brooks and E. M. Dunbar. MTP Press.

Your Notes and Questions

Tutorial 17: Allergies

Learning Objectives

1. **Natural History and Management Plans**
   - Allergic rhinitis
   - Allergic conjunctivitis
   - Food allergy
   - Milk allergy
   - Urticaria

2. **Indications for referral**

3. **Therapeutics**
   - Local therapy
   - Systemic therapy
   - Use of steroids
   - Elimination diets

4. **"Fringe medicine"**
   - Allergy clinics
   - Reflexologists

Skills

Prick Testing

Trainee Self Awareness

1. A 22 year old man arrives from France asking you to continue his course of desensitisation injections. How would you respond?
2. What is your management plan for hay fever? How would you deal with the acute severe problem, e.g. just before school examinations?
3. You are requested to refer a patient to an 'Allergy Clinic' because of claimed allergy due to beans and oranges. How would you respond?

Further Reading

ABC of Nutrition. BMJ Publications.

Your Notes and Questions

Tutorial 18: ENT Problems

Learning Objectives

1. **Natural History and Management Plans**
   Epistaxis
   Otitis Externa
   Otitis media - acute and recurrent
   Chronic serous otitis media
   Deafness in adults
   Deafness in children
   Tinnitus
   Vertigo - acute and chronic
   Hoarse voice
   Chronic catarrh and nasal obstruction

2. **Indications for referral**
   To whom

3. **Local referral for Hearing Aids**

4. **Services available to the hearing impaired**

5. **Role of routine audiograms and screening in the School Medical Service**

6. **Role and method of referral to Speech Therapists**

Skills

Otoscopy
Aural toilet and packing
Nasal packing and cautery for epistaxis
Interpretation of audiograms

Trainee Self Awareness

1. How might deafness present in early childhood? How can you help to minimise the possible adverse effects on a child's education?
2. What are your indications for referral of a child with chronic serous otitis media to an ENT surgeon? What treatment would you expect to be provided?
3. "He always has a cold, with a persistent blocked and runny nose". How would you manage this situation?
4. What help is available to the patient with persistent tinnitus?

Further Reading

ABC of ENT. BMJ Publications.
Common Diseases: their Nature, Incidence and Care. J. Fry. MTP Press.
Colour Atlas of Mouth, Throat and Ear Disorders. J. Bain et al. MTP Press.

Tutorial 19: Eyes

Learning Objectives

1. **Management of**
   - The Red Eye
   - Squint
   - Glaucoma
   - Sudden loss of vision
   - Gradual loss of vision
   - Internal and External Styes

2. **Role of the Optician**
   - Use of form GOS 18

3. **Screening Programmes and Methods for Glaucoma**

4. **Vision rules for driving**

5. **The Blind Register**
   - Criteria and benefits

Skills

Use of ophthalmoscope
Fluorescein staining
Everting upper lids and removal of foreign bodies
Cover test and squint detection
Use of Snellen and Near Vision Charts
Use of Ishihara Charts (Colour Vision)

Trainee Self Awareness

1. When should a red eye be referred for specialist opinion?
2. What constitutes an ophthalmic emergency? How would you go about arranging treatment in such an emergency?
3. "I think I have eye strain." How would you respond?
4. Glaucoma is a highly preventable cause of visual loss, yet it is still often diagnosed at a late stage. How can you improve your detection?

Further Reading
ABC of Ophthalmology. BMJ Publications.

Your Notes and Questions

Tutorial 20: Gastroenterology

Learning Objectives

1. **Natural History and Management Plans**
   - Oesophageal reflux and Hiatus Hernia
   - Peptic Ulcer
   - Non-Ulcer Dyspepsia
   - Irritable Bowel Syndrome
   - Diverticular Disease
   - Inflammatory Bowel Disease
   - Chronic Constipation
   - Pruritis Ani
   - Malignancy, including ostomy use
   - Haemorrhoids and Anal Fissure

2. **When to refer**
   - Surgeon?
   - Gastroenterologist (Physician)?

3. **Acute Problems**
   - Abdominal Pain
   - Haematemesis and Malaena
   - Diarrhoea and Vomiting

4. **Role of Specialist Stoma Nurses**

Skills

PR examination (rectal)
Proctoscopy

Trainee Self Awareness

1. Should GPs have direct access to investigations such as Gastroscopy and Barium Enema?
2. A 41 year old business executive asks for an H2 antagonist for his indigestion. He has had good relief after trying a colleague's tablets. How would you respond?
3. Should H2 antagonists be prescribed without definite diagnosis?
4. Would a practice management policy be of value in the management of gastro-enteritis. How would you plan it?

Further Reading

Gastroenterology. M. J. Lancaster-Smith and E. Chapman. MTP Press.

Your Notes and Questions

Tutorial 21: Epilepsy

Learning Objectives

1. **Natural History**
   - Grand mal
   - Petit mal
   - Focal: motor
     - sensory
     - temporal lobe
   - Febrile convulsions
   - Fits versus faints
   - Incidence and prevalence

2. **Management plans**
   - GP versus hospital in long term care
   - Drugs

3. **Management of an acute event**

4. **When to refer and to whom**

5. **Social and Psychological implications**
   - Occupation. Role of DRO (Disablement Resettlement Officer)
   - Education

6. **Self Help:**
   - British Epilepsy Association

7. **Rules for Driving**

Trainee Self Awareness

1. An epileptic on your list consults you having had two recent fits. You know he is continuing to drive. What do you do?
2. What are the indications for the measurement of serum anticonvulsant levels?
3. An 18 year old is newly diagnosed as epileptic. What problems is she likely to face?
4. Is lifelong treatment required for epilepsy?

Further Reading
Information folder on Epilepsy. RCGP Publications.
British Epilepsy Association, see Appendix 2.

Your Notes and Questions

Tutorial 22: Diabetes

Learning Objectives

1. **Natural History and Incidence**

2. **Management plan**
   Diet
   Oral Hypoglycaemic Drugs
   Insulin

3. **GP versus hospital care**

4. **When to refer**

5. **Intercurrent events such as**
   Pregnancy
   Infections e.g. respiratory, urinary and gastroenteritis

6. **Complications**

7. **Education**

8. **Self help groups:** British Diabetic Association

9. **Health care team**
   Dietician
   Chiropodist
   Ophthalmologist and Optician
   Diabetic Liaison Nurse

10. **Management of acute problems**

11. **Rules for driving**

Skills

Use of Glucometer
Examination of fundi and feet

Trainee Self Awareness

1. Formulate a practice policy for the follow up of diabetics.
2. There is debate as to whether good control reduces long term complications. What is your opinion?
3. Discuss the role of a mini-clinic versus opportunistic review.
4. What problems might face a new diabetic? Consider the case of a 15 year old and a 76 year old.

Further Reading
ABC of Diabetes. BMJ Publications.
Information folder on Diabetes. RCGP Publications.
British Diabetic Association, see Appendix 2.

Your Notes and Questions

Tutorial 23: Upper Respiratory Tract Infection

Learning Objectives

1. **Natural History**
   Common cold
   Sinusitis
   Sore throat
   Tonsillitis
   Otitis media
   Croup

2. **Management Plans of above Common Diseases**
   Therapy: symptomatic
   indications for use of antibiotics
   Indications for further investigation

3. **Indications for referral**

4. **The 'Catarrhal Child Syndrome'**

Trainee Self Awareness

1. What are your indications for treating a sore throat with an antibiotic? What factors influence your decision?
2. When would you admit a child with croup to hospital?
3. What may lead to a request for tonsillectomy from a patient or parent? What are your indications for referral for this operation?
4. Do you have a preferred antibiotic regime for the treatment of otitis media? What factors influence your choice?

Further Reading

ABC of ENT. BMJ Publications.
Common Diseases: their Nature, Incidence and Care. J. Fry. MTP Press.

Your Notes and Questions

Tutorial 24: Chronic Obstructive Airways Disease (COAD)

Learning Objectives

1. **Natural History:**
    - Chronic Bronchitis
    - Emphysema

2. **Management**
    - Drugs:
        - Bronchodilators: range of inhaled drugs and devices; oral preparations
        - Steroids
        - Antibiotics
    - Oxygen:
        - Indications
        - Prescriptions
        - Oxygen concentrators
    - Role of Nebulisers
    - Physiotherapy

3. **Social Support**

4. **Acute exacerbations:** home versus hospital

5. **Indications for referral**

6. **Long term management plan** (Planned care approach)

Skills

Use of Peak Flow Meter
Use of Inhalers and Nebulisers
Prescription of Oxygen and Oxygen Concentrators

Trainee Self Awareness

1. A patient has been severely disabled by COAD, and has been deteriorating for some time. A CXR shows a large hilar mass suggestive of malignancy. How would you manage the problem?
2. A patient is told by the hospital that he would benefit from domiciliary oxygen. He lives alone in a block of flats, and you know he continues to smoke. How do you respond to his request to arrange it?
3. A patient asks for oxygen at home as she is sure it will make her feel better. What is your response?
4. A patient who is using inhaled steroids has recurrent oral thrush. What is your short term and long term management?

Further Reading

Drug Tariff Supply of Oxygen. DHSS.

Tutorial 25: Asthma

Learning Objectives

1. **Knowledge of Natural History and Management**
   Adults
   Children

2. **Management Plans**
   A. Symptomatic: brochodilators
   theophyllines
   B. Preventative: disodium cromoglycate
   inhaled steroids
   C. Acute Emergencies

3. **Use of:**
   Steroids
   Antibiotics
   Nebulisers

4. **Indications for acute admissions**

5. **Special problems:**
   Young children, less than 2 years old
   Brittle asthmatics
   Chronic cough and night cough

6. **Patient involvement:**
   Self monitoring and medication
   Asthma Society
   Special diets

Skills

Use of Peak Flow Meters
Ability to demonstrate correct use of inhaler technique
Use of nebulisers

Trainee Self Awareness

1. Despite advances in treatment of asthma, the mortality rate from asthma has not dramatically fallen. What reasons may account for this fact?
2. How would you assess the degree of control of a patient's asthma?
3. What are the advantages, and disadvantages, of an asthmatic patient's referral to a hospital clinic?
4. What would you say to the mother of a 3 year old child whom you have just diagnosed as having asthma? What might be the mother's reaction?

Further Reading

ABC of Asthma. BMJ Publications.
Practical Management of Asthma. T. Clark and J. Rees. Dunitz.
Information folder on Asthma. RCGP Publications.
Asthma Society, see Appendix 2.

Your Notes and Questions

Tutorial 26: Ischaemic Heart Disease

Learning Objectives

1. **Knowledge of Natural History and Epidemiology**

2. **Risk Factor Identification**
   Screening

3. **Risk Factor Modification**
   Health Education
   Non-drug methods
   Drug methods

4. **Management of Hyperlipidaemia**

5. **Angina**
   Management Plan: stepped care drug approach
   Indications for referral

6. **Myocardial Infarction**
   Acute management: hospital versus home management
   Post infarction management: cardiac rehabilitation

7. **Cardiac Surgery**
   Coronary artery bypass grafting and angioplasty
      Indications
      Postoperative management

8. **Rules for Driving, including HGV and PSV**

9. **Management of 'Chest Pain'**

Skills

Reading and taking ECG

Trainee Self Awareness

1. Discuss the advantages and disadvantages of the practice owning its own ECG machine
2. Describe how you could organise your practice to increase the detection of cardio-vascular disease risk factors. What is the place of delegation to other members of the Primary Health Care Team?
3. What are your indications for referral of patients suffering from angina?
4. What role do you play in helping patients to give up smoking? Outline your management approach.

Further Reading:
Practising Prevention. BMJ Publications.
Prevention of Coronary Heart Disease and Stroke. A Workbook for Primary Health Care Teams. J. T. Hart and B. Stilwell. Faber and Faber.

Your Notes and Questions

Tutorial 27: Hypertension

Learning Objectives

1. **Natural History and Epidemiology**

2. **Management Plan**
   Identification and Evaluation
   Non drug treatment
   Drug therapy
   Principles of stepped-care approach
   Associated risk factor management
   Evaluation of end organ damage

3. **Long term follow up plan**
   What investigations and why

4. **Indications for referral**
   To whom: General Physician
   Cardiologist
   Renal Physician

5. **Management in special categories**
   Young
   Old
   Systolic only
   Concurrent illness: Diabetes
   Asthma

6. **Knowledge of Therapeutic agents**
   Indication
   Action
   Side effects

7. **Results of Hypertension Trials**
   e.g. MRC (Medical Research Council)
   EWPHE (European Working Party in Hypertension in the Elderly)
   What level should one treat?
   What other lessons are to be learned?

8. **Screening for Hypertension**
   Systematic versus opportunistic
   Role of Practice nurse
   Record systems for optimum care

Skills

Use of sphygmomanometer

Trainee Self Awareness

1. How may patients with hypertension present? What are the implications for the Primary Health Care Team
2. What investigations do you routinely perform on your hypertensive patients? Why do you do this?
3. How may poor compliance and side effects of anti-hypertensive drugs be reduced?
4. What do you regard as optimum care for your hypertensive patient? How can you achieve this?

Further Reading

ABC of Hypertension. BMJ Publications.
Blood Pressure Measurement. BMJ Publications.
Hypertension. J. Tudor Hart. Library of General Practice. Churchill Livingstone.

Your Notes and Questions

Tutorial 28: Cerebrovascular Disease

Learning Objectives

1. **Natural History and Definitions**
   e.g. Transient Ischaemic Attacks (TIA)
   Incidence

2. **Risk Factors and Prevention**

3. **Prognosis**

4. **Acute Management**
   Indications for referral
   Home versus hospital
   Support available

5. **Investigations**

6. **Long Term Management**
   Role of primary health care team
   Physiotherapy and occupational therapy
   Support systems for patients and carers
   Long term problems

7. **Provision of aids**
   Personal nursing aids
   Home adaption and aids to daily living (ADL)
   Wheelchairs: ALAC form

Trainee Self Awareness

1. What problems would a 76 year old widow face following a CVA?
2. A 34 year old man has a Subarachnoid Haemorrhage. What facilities for rehabilitation are available, and what are the implications for him and his family?
3. The wife of a 60 year old stroke patient is caring for him at home. She threatens to kill herself and her husband as "life is not worth living". What action would you take?

Further Reading
Everyday Aids and Appliances. BMJ Publications.
Information Folder on Parkinson's Disease. RCGP Publications.
Association of Carers, see Appendix 2.

Your Notes and Questions

Tutorial 29: Joint Problems

Learning Objectives

1. **Natural History**
   - Gout
   - Acute Arthritis, including Injuries
   - Chronic Arthritis
   - Knee Problems, Acute and Chronic
   - Shoulder Problems
   - Tendinoses

2. **Investigations**

3. **Management**
   - Drugs
   - Rest and/or specific exercises
   - Physiotherapy - methods of local referral
   - Injections

4. **Referral**
   - To Whom

Skills

Joint Aspiration
Injection Technique
  Tennis/Golfer's Elbow
  Shoulder

Trainee Self Awareness

1. A 14 year old girl presents with a painful knee. What is the differential diagnosis, and how would you manage the problem?
2. A 40 year old woman presents with a 2 week history of a painful shoulder. How do you treat her?
3. What are your indications for the prophylaxis of gout?
4. Many patients are on long term anti-inflammatory drugs. What are the problems produced by this?

Further Reading

ABC of Practical Procedures. BMJ Publications.
Locomotor Disability in General Practice. M. I. V. Jayson and R. Million. Oxford University Press.

Your Notes and Questions

Tutorial 30: Back and Neck Pain

Learning Objectives

1. **Back Pain**
   - Causes: Unknown (the majority)
     - Prolapsed Intervertebral Disc
     - Spondylitis
   - Examination
   - Investigations

2. **Treatment:** Acute attack
   - Chronic pain
     - Drugs
     - Rest
     - Physiotherapy
     - Chiropracter
     - Osteopath
     - Traction
     - Surgery
     - Indications for referral: Orthopaedic Surgeon, Neurosurgeon, Rheumatologist

3. **Neck Pain**
   - Causes
   - Whiplash Injuries
   - Management and Prognosis
   - Treatment as above
   - Use of Collars
   - Use of Accident and Emergency services

4. **Consider contribution of underlying psychological problem.**

Trainee Self Awareness

1. You have been treating a 44 year old with back pain for some time. He asks for another sick note but you are not sure he has enough of a problem to warrant it. How do you respond?
2. Should General Practitioners have access to physiotherapy services?
3. What is the incidence of spondylitis? How can we help early diagnosis?
4. Could Health Education reduce the incidence of Back Pain?

Further Reading

Locomotor Disability in General Practice. M. I. V. Jayson and R. Million. Oxford University Press.

Your Notes and Questions

Tutorial 31: UTI and Prostatism

Learning Objectives

1. **Natural History and Management Plans for UTI**
   - Children
   - Women
   - Men
   - Recurrent
   - Pregnancy
   - Asymptomatic Bacteriuria

2. **Significance of MSU**

3. **Referral**
   - When
   - To whom

4. **Prostatism**
   - Natural History
   - When to refer

5. **Urethral Syndrome**

Skills

Bedside Microscopy

Trainee Self Awareness

1. How useful is an MSU? Does it alter management?
2. How useful are 'self help' measures in the management of cystitis?
3. A 69 year old man is on the waiting list for prostatectomy. He asks you if it will affect his sexual function. How do you respond?
4. How would you manage an 11 year old boy who presents with enuresis?

Further Reading

Urology: Library of General Practice. D. Brooks and N. Mallick. Churchill Livingstone.
An Atlas of Bedside Microscopy. Occasional Paper 32. RCGP Publications.

Your Notes and Questions

Tutorial 32: Antenatal Care

Learning Objectives

1. **Schedule of Care**
   Booking procedure
   Antenatal visits
   Intrapartum care
   Postnatal care

2. **Concept of Obstetric List**

3. **Regulations and Obligations of care.** See SFA 31

4. **Ability to Identify problems, e.g.** PET (Pre-Eclamptic Toxaemia), IUGR (Intrauterine Growth Retardation)

5. **Role and Obligations of the Midwife**

6. **Social Aspects**
   Role of Health Visitor, Social Worker, Benefits, and Antenatal and Parentcraft classes

7. **Psychological problems e.g.** fears, early identification of depression

8. **Drugs in pregnancy**

9. **Forms:**

Booking:	FP24/FP24 A (obstetric list/not on obstetric list) Claim form for medical services. Should be signed by patient at booking. Complete after postnatal examination and forward to FPC for payment.
	FW 8 Certificate of Pregnancy. Signed by Medical Practitioner, Midwife or Health Visitor. Completed and sent by patient to FPC to obtain certificate for free prescriptions etc.
26th week:	MAT B1 Certificate of Expected Confinement. Needed to claim statutory maternity pay and maternity benefits.
Postnatal:	Complete FP24. Record each postnatal visit. (Maximum 5 visits up to 14 days post partum). Postnatal examination before 12 weeks to claim fee. Submit claim within 6 months.
	Contraception: FP1001 or FP 1002 Cervical smear: FP 74

Skills

Use of Sonicaid

Use of Kick Chart
Episiotomy repair

Trainee Self Awareness

1. One of your patients is insistent she wants a home delivery. How do you advise her and what are your obligations?
2. What patients would you book and what procedures would you undertake on a GP unit? What do you see as the advantages and disadvantages?
3. What are your views on the midwife's role as a sole practitioner?
4. A 33 year old patient in her first pregnancy is a keen member of the National Childbirth Trust (NCT). How do you respond to her request for "no intervention"?

Further Reading

SFA (The Red Book) paragraph 31. Family Practitioner Committee.
Booking for Maternity Care, A Comparison of Two Systems. Occasional Paper 31. RCGP Publications.
Notes for the DRCOG. P. Kaye. Churchill Livingstone.

Your Notes and Questions

Tutorial 33: Premenstrual Syndrome

Learning Objectives

1. Natural History
- Nature and timing of symptoms
- Concept of symptom free days
- Initiating factors
- Theories on aetiology

2. Treatment Plan
- Psychological
  - Self Help
  - Counselling
- Physical
  - Exercise
  - Diet
- Drugs
  - Non Hormonal
  - Hormonal
- Health Education

Skills

Use of a Symptom Diary

Trainee Self Awareness

1. A patient complains of severe Premenstrual Tension (PMT). How would you assess the best treatment plan?
2. A 35 year old woman who has been seen by you with premenstrual symptoms is caught shoplifting. She asks you for medical defence of her action. What do you do?
3. A patient asks you whether you think she should try Oil of Evening Primrose for PMT. How do you respond?
4. There has been an increasing number of presentations with PMT. Does this reflect an increasing incidence or increased awareness? Have we been guilty of not previously giving symptoms due respect?

Further Reading

Women's Problems in General Practice. A. McPherson and A. Anderson. Oxford University Press.

Notes for the DRCOG. P. Kaye. Churchill Livingstone.

Your Notes and Questions

Tutorial 34: Cervix

Learning Objectives

1. **Natural History of Cervical Abnormalities**

2. **Risk Factors**

3. **Cervical Screening Programmes**
   Principles
   Effect of programme
   Practice system
   Local system
   Call and recall
   Follow up of abnormalities

4. **Management of the abnormal smear**
   Implications of abnormalities
   Indications for referral
   Use of colposcopy

5. **Health Education**

6. **Forms**
   FP74 Cervical cytology claim.
   Fee payable for the first smear after age 35 or 3 pregnancies, then for first testing in each 5 year period where the patient's age ends in 5 or 0.

7. **Rules for Payments for repeat smears**

Skills

Taking a cervical smear
Setting up a screening programme

Trainee Self Awareness

1. Screening for cancer of the cervix in England has not reduced mortality from the disease, although it has in Iceland. What factors may account for this?
2. A smear taken during pregnancy is reported as 'Inflammatory changes with moderate dyskariosis'. What are the implications of this?
3. How do you ensure a complete follow up of abnormal smear reports?
4. What advice can you give a 17 year old to help prevent cervical carcinoma? When and how might you provide this advice?

Further Reading

SFA (The Red Book) Paragraph 28. Family Practitioner Committee.
Women's problems in General Practice. A. McPherson and A. Anderson. Oxford University Press.
Information Folder on Cervical Cytology. RCGP Publications.

Tutorial 35: Family Planning

Learning Objectives

1. **Methods Available**
   - Natural
   - Barrier
   - IUCD
   - Hormonal
   - Surgical
   - Post coital
   - T.O.P. (Termination of Pregnancy)

2. **Special Categories**
   - Young
   - Over 40s
   - Medical Problems, e.g. hypertension
diabetes
epilepsy

3. **GP Care versus Family Planning Clinic**

4. **Legal Aspects.** Abortion Act 1967.

5. **JCC Certificate.** Training required.

6. **Forms**
   - Record Cards
   - FP1001 contraceptive services
   - FP1002 intrauterine device
   - FP1003 contraception for a temporary resident
   - HSA1 abortion certificate

Skills

Cap fitting
IUCD insertion

Trainee Self Awareness

1. A 40 year old non-smoker asks to go on the pill. What is your response?
2. Compare the morbidity and mortality for a healthy 43 year old between oral contraception and a tubal ligation.
3. A 15 year old asks to go on the pill. How do you counsel her?
4. A single woman presents 48 hours after unprotected intercourse. What treatment can you offer? What follow up is required?
5. How would you counsel the mother of a mentally retarded 19 year old girl concerning contraception for her daughter.
6. What are the legal grounds for performing a T.O.P. under the Abortion Act 1967?

Further Reading

Handbook of Contraceptive Practice. DHSS.
Contraceptive Practice. M. Potts and P. Diggory. Cambridge University Press.
SFA (The Red Book) Paragraph 29. Family Practitioner Committee.

J.C.C. Certificate Requirements: details from Joint Committee on Contraception. c/o Royal College of Obstetricians and Gynaecologists, 27 Sussex Place, London NW1 4RG. (Tel: 01-262 5425)

Your Notes and Questions

Tutorial 36: Menopause

Learning Objectives

1. **Range of Problems**
   - Gynaecological
     - local
     - sexual
     - contraception
   - Cardiovascular
   - Psychological
   - Osteoporosis

2. **Management**
   - Aims of treatment: e.g. Relief of symptoms
     Prevention of osteoporosis

3. **Drugs**
   - Non hormonal
   - Hormonal(HRT)
     - Benefit versus risk
     - Length of treatment
     - Role of progestogens
     - Cost effectiveness
     - Contraindications
   - Local Hormonal treatment

4. **Self Help Groups**

5. **Patient literature**

6. **Psychological aspects**

7. **Indications for referral**

Trainee Self Awareness

1. An attractive young looking 50 year old asks for 'hormone treatment'. What is your reaction?
2. 'We should treat all menopausal patients with HRT'. Discuss.
3. A menopausal patient suffers with severe hot flushes. HRT is contraindicated due to a previous mastectomy. What help can you offer?
4. A 52 year old woman has not had a period for 12 months. She asks you what she should do regarding contraception. What advice would you give?

Further Reading

Women's Problems in General Practice. A. McPherson and A. Anderson. Oxford University Press.

The Menopause. J. Coope. BMA Family Doctor Publications.

Tutorial 37: Infertility

Learning Objectives

1. Incidence

2. Causes

3. 'Average' time to conception

4. Management Plan Semen analysis
Assess ovulation
21 day progesterone
Role of temperature charts
Use of clomiphene
When and whom to refer

5. Current methods of intervention and success rate

6. Psychological effects of infertility

Skills

Post coital test

Trainee Self Awareness

1. A 34 year old woman presents with a 6 month history of infertility. What is your response and subsequent action?
2. A 27 year old woman presents with 3 years infertility. She tells you that her husband refuses to see you about the matter. What help can you give her?
3. A woman of 38 years old asks for referral to a private infertility agency. What is your response?
4. A married couple in their thirties present, very pleased about a positive pregnancy test. Investigations by you had shown the husband to be azoospermic. What is your response?
5. What problems might a couple face who have conceived by AID (Artificial Insemination by Donor)?

Further Reading

Notes for the DRCOG. P. Kaye. Churchill Livingstone.
Womens Problems in General Practice. A. McPherson and A. Anderson. Oxford University Press.

Tutorial 38: Vaginal Discharge

Learning Objectives

1. **Causes**
   Commonly Candida, Trichomonas and Gardnerella
   Remember Sexually Transmitted Diseases (see Tutorial 40)
   Remember Foreign Bodies

2. **Investigation**
   When and How

3. **Treatment**
   Regime
   When to treat partner

4. **Referral**
   Gynaecologist
   STD Clinic

5. **Vaginal discharge in children**
   Management
   Possibility of sexual abuse

6. **Concept of underlying psycho-sexual problems,** presenting as vaginal discharge

Skills

Vaginal examination. Use of speculum
Swab taking - HVS, Cervical
Bedside microscopy
Minor procedures, e.g. Removal of polyp

Trainee Self Awareness

1. A 28 year old woman presents with a vaginal discharge which proves to be associated with a chlamydial infection. She asks if she could have caught it from her husband. What is your reply?
2. A 63 year old postmenopausal woman presents with an episode of post coital bleeding. On examination you find and remove a cervical polyp. Is any further action required?
3. A 19 year old has been treated for a candidal infection. She asks you for a supply of pessaries to keep 'in stock'. What is your reaction?
4. An anxious 22 year old, recently married, complains of an unpleasant discharge after intercourse. She is convinced that she has an infection. How do you manage the problem?

Further Reading

Women's Problems in General Practice. A. McPherson and A. Anderson. Oxford University Press.

An Atlas of Bedside Microscopy. Occasional Paper 32 (1986). RCGP Publications.

Your Notes and Questions

Tutorial 39: Abnormal Vaginal Bleeding

Learning Objectives

1. **Causes and Management Plan**
   - Threatened Miscarriage
   - Ectopic Pregnancy
   - Dysfunctional Uterine Bleeding
   - Progesterone only pill
   - IUCD
   - Pelvic inflammatory disease
   - Carcinoma
   - Local causes, e.g. polyp, atrophy
   - Menorrhagia
2. **Acute Problem**
   - Life threatening blood loss
3. **Indication for referral**
4. **Principles of Therapeutics**
   - Non-hormonal
   - Hormonal

Skills

Vaginal Examination

Trainee Self Awareness

1. You are called to the house of a 28 year old woman who is bleeding vaginally and is clinically shocked. What do you do?
2. A 70 year old woman has noticed some vaginal spotting. Examination reveals an atrophic epithelium. How do you treat her?
3. Discuss the problems of a 25 year old woman who has been discharged from hospital following a miscarriage.
4. What are your indications for a D and C for a patient on HRT therapy?
5. Should GPs have open access to ultrasound scan facilities?

Further Reading

Women's Problems in General Practice. A. McPherson and A. Anderson. Oxford University Press.

Notes for the DRCOG. P. Kaye. Churchill Livingstone.

Your Notes and Questions

Tutorial 40: Sexually Transmitted Diseases and AIDS

Learning Objectives

1. **Range of Infections**
   Bacterial, fungal, protozoal, viral

2. **Diagnosis**

3. **Treatment: Implications if not treated**

4. **Contact tracing**

5. **Role of special clinics** (STD Clinics)

6. **Acquired Immune Deficiency Syndrome** (AIDS)
   Epidemiology
   Natural history
   Clinical features
   Management and prognosis
   Implications of a positive HIV test
   Pre and post test counselling. The role of an AIDS counsellor
   Health Education and Prevention

Skills

Swab taking
Microscopy

Trainee Self Awareness

1. A businessman returns from a trip abroad and presents with a penile discharge. He refuses to attend a STD clinic and demands that you do not tell his wife. What are the implications?
2. Should STD clinics inform GP's of their investigations and treatment, including AIDS?
3. Should all patients with Trichomonas vaginalis be referred for serology?
4. You are sent an insurance proposal form to complete. There is a question asking "Is this patient at risk of contracting AIDS"? Your patient has had HIV testing following an affair, but asks you not to mention it. What do you do?
5. Should we ever test for AIDS without consent?

Further Reading

Women's Problems in General Practice. A. McPherson and A. Anderson. Oxford University Press.
An Atlas of Bedside Microscopy. Occassional Paper 32. RCGP Publications.
ABC of Sexually Transmitted Diseases. BMJ Publications.
ABC of AIDS. BMJ Publications.
Terence Higgins Trust, see Appendix 2.

Tutorial 41: Development Checks

Learning Objectives

1. **Best ages for assessment**

2. **Procedure taken**
   General history
   Developmental history
   Physical examination
   Growth check
   Motor development
   Social responses
   Vocalisation
   Vision
   Hearing

3. **Interpretation of Abnormalities**
   Range of normal
   Significance of prematurity
   Emotional deprivation
   Mental subnormality
   Hearing/visual loss
   Autism

Trainee Self Awareness

1. Who should carry out developmental checks? GP, Health visitor or Clinical Medical Officer.
2. The parents of a 6 month old baby are worried that he cannot hear. What can you do?
3. What do you consider to be the best ages for carrying out checks?

Further Reading

Basic Developmental Screening 0-4 years. R. S. Illingworth. Churchill Livingstone.
ABC of 1-7. BMJ Publications.

Your Notes and Questions

Tutorial 42: Feeding Problems in Infants

Learning Objectives

1. **Normal feeding regimes** e.g. Bottle feeding requirements 0-4 months is 150 ml/kg/day.
    Breast feeding versus bottle feeding
    Vitamin and mineral supplements
    Introduction of solids
    Milk allergy
    Lactose intolerance
    Toddler's diarrhoea

2. **Management Plan for Problems**
    Colic
    Reflux
    Gastroenteritis

Skills

Feeding techniques
Percentile charts

Trainee Self Awareness

1. A new mother consults you. She says her Health Visitor is concerned about her breast fed baby's weight gain. The weight is on the 15th percentile. She asks you if she should change to bottle feeds. How would you respond?
2. A mother asks you for a prescription for soya milk. She tells you that her baby vomits after every feed, and she is sure he is allergic to his milk. What do you do?
3. A three month old baby has recently recovered from gastroenteritis. Mum says he must have relapsed as his stools are watery. What advice do you give?
4. A breast feeding mother develops a tender red triangle on one breast. How do you manage the problem?

Further reading

A Paediatric Vade-Mecum. J. Insley and B. Wood. LLoyd Luke.
ABC of Nutrition. BMJ Publications.
The Normal Child. R. S. Illingworth. Churchill Livingstone.

Your Notes and Questions

Tutorial 43: Child Abuse

Learning Objectives

1. **Clinical Features of non-accidental injury and sexual abuse**

2. **Predisposing factors**
   Social
   Family

3. **Presentation**
   Becoming alerted to the possibility

4. **Management Plan**
   Local referral plan
   Health Visitors
   Notification to Social Services
   Consultant Paediatrician
   Case Conference
   Place of Safety Order. Responsibility of Social Services
   Role of other agencies
   NSPCC

Skills

Preparation of medico-legal reports
Principles of consent and confidentiality
Family support

Trainee Self Awareness

1. What is the 'at risk' register? How might the GP be involved in the prevention of child abuse?
2. What is the value of the Case Conference? Who should be present and what is your role?
3. When should a child be taken compulsorily into the care of the Local Authority? How might this be arranged?
4. You suspect sexual abuse in a 7 year old girl. What is your management plan?

Further Reading
Commonsense Paediatrics. M. Pollak and J. Fry. MTP Press.

Your Notes and Questions

Tutorial 44: Immunisation

Learning Objectives

1. **Programmes Available**

   Diphtheria, Pertussis, Tetanus } DPT

   Measles, Mumps, Rubella } MMR

   Polio

   BCG
   Hepatitis B
   Influenza

2. **Basis of Immunisation**

   Indications and contraindications

3. **Local Immunisation programme**

4. **Own practice versus DHA run clinic**

5. **Dispensing own vaccines**: See SFA 44

6. **Assessing uptake**

   Recall facilities

7. **Role of Health Visitor and Practice Nurse**

8. **Domicilliary immunisations for special risk groups**

9. **Forms**

   FP 73 Vaccination and Immunisation Claim Form
   FP 7A (male), FP 8A (female). Vaccination and Immunisation record cards

Trainee Self Awareness

1. A mother is worried about having her baby immunised against whooping cough. How would you advise her?
2. A 6 month old baby has not yet been immunised because he was 'snuffly' at each clinic attendance. What would you do?
3. A pregnant mother comes in contact with rubella. What is your action?
   You have recently immunised a 17 year old girl against rubella. She is pregnant. What do you do.

Further Reading

SFA (The Red Book) paragraph 27. Family Practitioner Committee.
Immunisation against Infectious Disease. DHSS.

Tutorial 45: Overseas Travel and Immunisation/Vaccination

Learning Objectives

1. **Use of and contraindications to:**
   Cholera
   Typhoid
   Polio
   Yellow fever
   Gammaglobulin

2. **Immunisation programme**

3. **Effectiveness of vaccination**

4. **Malaria prophylaxis**

5. **General advice**

6. **Contraindications to flying**

7. **Forms**
   FP 73 Vaccination and Immunisation Claim Form
   CH 7 AHA unscheduled attendances. Accepted by some FPC for adult and foreign travel immunisation

   International Certificate of Vaccination against Cholera and Typhoid

   Other Immunisation Certificates: not standard

Trainee Self Awareness

1. A family with 3 children aged 6 months, 2 years and 12 years are going to Bali for a holiday. What immunisation programme would you arrange?
2. A student asks for the necessary immunisations as he is going to India in two weeks time. What do you suggest?
3. A woman who is 35 weeks pregnant asks if she can fly over to Ireland to stay with her family. What is your advice?

Further Reading

ABC of Healthy Travel. BMJ Publications.
SFA (The Red Book) Paragraph 27. Family Practitioner Committee.

Advice Centres:

England

1. International Relations, (Health) Branch, DHSS, Alexander Fleming House, Elephant and Castle, London SE1 6BY. Tel: 01 407 5522 extensions 6749, 6711.
2. Public Health Laboratory Service, Communicable Disease Surveillance Centre, 61 Colindale Avenue, London NW9 5EQ. Tel: 01 200 6868.

Wales

3. DHSS Welsh Office, Cathays Park, Cardiff CF1 3NQ. Tel: Cardiff 825111 extension 3336.

Scotland

4. Scottish Home and Health Department, St Andrew's House, Edinburgh EH1 3DE. Tel: Edinburgh (031) 5568501 extension 2438.
   or for vaccination information only:
5. The Communicable Diseases (Scotland) Unit, Ruchill Hospital, Bilsland Drive, Glasgow G20 9NB. Tel: Glasgow (041) 9467120.

Northern Ireland

6. DHSS Dundonald House, Upper Newtownards Road, Belfast BT4 3SF. Tel: Belfast 63939 extension 2593.

Malaria Advice

Malaria Reference Laboratory, London School of Hygiene and Tropical Medicine, Keppel Street, London WC1E 7HT. Tel: 01 636 7921.

Your Notes and Questions

Tutorial 46: Geriatrics

15% of the present population are over 65 years of age.

Learning Objectives

1. **'Normal Ageing Process'** and its associated physical, psychological and social consequences.

2. **Common Problems**
   - Falls
   - Weight loss
   - Dementia/Depression
   - Hypothermia
   - Heart Failure
   - Parkinsonism
   - Polymyalgia

3. **Practical Assessment in the Home**
   - Can they communicate?
     - deafness, vision
   - Can they get out and about?
     - arthritis
     - painful feet
     - walking sticks/frame
   - Can they look after themselves?
     - dressing
     - washing and cleaning
     - feeding and cooking
     - laundry
     - confidence
   - Are they safe?
     - at risk from hypothermia?
   - Are they taking the right medication?
     - clear instructions
     - is the drug really necessary
     - is the medicine in the easiest dose regime
   - Are they lonely?
     - is support available?
   - What about the carers?

4. **Support services**

   GP

   Statutory: (1) District Medical Services

   Nursing services: HV, DN, Bath Nurse
   Audiology (hearing aids)
   Chiropody
   Physiotherapy and Occupational Therapy

Geriatric Unit Admission - Long and short-term care:
Day Hospital
Domiciliary Geriatric Visit

Psychiatry

(2) Social Services
Social Worker, Home Help, Meals on Wheels, Day Centre

Voluntary: OAP Clubs, Age Concern

5. Residential Care

Warden controlled flats (sheltered housing)
Elderly Persons Home (Part III accommodation)
Rest Home/Nursing Homes

6. Geriatric Screening

7. 'At Risk' Registers

Trainee Self Awareness

1. Discuss the problems of keeping the elderly in their relative's homes.
2. How can the Primary Health Care team establish a policy for the care of the elderly in the practice?
3. How do you respond to "She's getting too much for me with all these falls. She'll have to be put away"? What are your options?
4. How may repeat prescriptions be hazardous to the elderly patient? How can this be prevented?

Further Reading

Preventative Care of the Elderly. A review of Current Developments. Occasional Paper 25. RCGP Publications.

Lecture Notes on Geriatrics. N. Coni. W. Davison and S. Webster. Blackwell Scientific Publications.

Medicine in Old Age. BMJ Publications.

Your Notes and Questions

Tutorial 47: Terminal Care

Learning Objectives

1. **Management Plan for terminal care in general practice**
   - Physical
     - pain relief
     - other symptom relief
     - use of opiates, including injection pump
   - Psychological
   - Spiritual
   - Social
   - Relatives and Carers

2. **Terminal Care Team Concept**
   Roles and referral method:
   - Community (district) nurse
   - Health Visitor
   - Marie Curie nurses
   - Macmillan nurses
   - Hospice Community Team

3. **Hospice versus Home Management**

4. **Stages of dying** (after Kubler Ross)
   - Denial
   - Anger
   - Bargaining
   - Depression
   - Acceptance

Skills

Versatility of therapeutic options
Team work

Trainee Self Awareness

1. What are the emotional needs of the dying and their relatives? How can they be met?
2. What are your indications for admission to a Hospice?
3. Terminal care is emotionally demanding on the doctor and the primary health care team. Discuss how this can be coped with.
4. How could you assess the effectiveness of the care your practice gives to the dying patient?

Further Reading

Terminal Care. R. Spilling. Oxford University Press.

Tutorial 48: Bereavement

Learning Objectives

1. **Normal phases of Mourning** (after Colin Murray Parkes)
   - Numbness
   - Yearning and Anger
   - Disorganisation and Despair
   - Restitution (mourning can take 1-2 years)

2. **Tasks of Mourning** (after Worden)
   - Accept the reality of the loss
   - Experience the pain of grief
   - Adjust to the environment in which the deceased is missing
   - Reinvest emotional energy into other relationships. (Endpoint of mourning)

3. **Factors affecting grief**
   - Closeness of relationship
   - Living alone
   - Lack of support
   - Sudden death
   - Death of a child

4. **Management of Normal Grief**
   - Provide continuing support
   - Provide time to grieve
   - Allow expression of emotions and stay with them
   - Reassurance of normality of reaction:
     - Feelings: sadness/anger/guilt/helplessness
     - Physical sensations: 'hollow in the stomach'/tight throat/sighing
     - Thoughts: disbelief/confusion/sense of presence/hallucinations
     - Behaviour: sleep disturbance/dreams/searching/looking for reminders of the deceased
   - Work through the Tasks of Mourning
   - Consider medication

5. **Abnormal Grief Response**
   - Complicated Grief: failure/chronic/delayed/exaggerated/masked
   - Anticipated Grief
   - Grief under special circumstances: suicide/abortion/sudden death/cot death stillbirth

6. **Support Systems**
   - Clergy/voluntary e.g. CRUSE

Trainee Self Awareness

1. Own experience of grief. Is this affecting your outlook? Increased sensitivity to own personal death awareness. Coping with the emotions and behaviour of the newly bereaved.

2. What is the importance of the normal grief reaction?
3. What is the GP's role in the follow up of the newly bereaved? How long would you provide follow up?
4. What are the indications for sedatives and anti-depressants in the bereaved?
5. What support systems are available during mourning of the bereaved?
6. An urgent call is requested to a mother who has found her 3 month old baby dead in it's cot.
   What immediate reactions might you anticipate in the mother?
   Why might guilt feelings be so strong?
   What would you do immediately?
   What are common reactions of friends and relatives to the parents?
   What advice would you give about another pregnancy?

Further Reading

Grief Counselling and Grief Therapy. W. Worden. Tavistock Publications.
Cruse, see Appendix 2.
Cot Death Research and Support Associations, see Appendix 2.

Your Notes and Questions

Tutorial 49: Audit and Research

Learning Objectives

1. The concept of achieving 'Quality in General Practice'.
How may this be measured?

2. The methods and difficulties of performing a practice Audit.

3. The methodology of setting up a practice research project.

4. The use of audit as a method of assessment and continuing medical education.

Trainee Self Awareness

1. Consider a small project, audit or research.
2. What is meant by the terms 'Process, Structure and Outcome'?
3. What is involved in a 'What Sort of Doctor' assessment?

Further Reading
Research and General Practice. J. Howie. Croom Helm.
In Pursuit of Quality. RCGP Publications.
Quality in General Practice (1985). Policy Statement 2. RCGP Publications.
What sort of Doctor? (1985). Reports from General Practice 23. RCGP Publications.
Medical Audit in General Practice (1982). Occasional Paper 20. RCGP Publications.
Trainee Projects (1985). Occasional Paper 29. RCGP Publications.

Your Notes and Questions

Tutorial 50: Patients and the General Practitioner

Learning Objectives

1. **Self Help Groups** (see Appendix 1)

2. **Patient Participation Groups** (PPG)

3. **Community Health Council** (CHC)

4. **Practising Medicine in Different Areas**
   Inner City
   Rural

5. **Transcultural medicine**

6. **Well Women Clinics**

Trainee Self Awareness

1. What difficulties may arise in consultations when doctor and patient have different cultural backgrounds?
2. What is the value of self help groups?
3. How do you respond to the patient who disagrees with your opinion? How can you resolve this problem?
4. Some practices have formed PPG's. What might their aim be?

Further Reading

Patient Participation in General Practice (1981). Occasional Paper 17. RCGP Publications.
Inner Cities (1982). Occasional Paper 19. RCGP Publications.
Social Class and Health Status. Inequality or Difference (1984). Occasional Paper 25. RCGP Publications.
Medical Practice in a Multicultural Society. Fuller and Toon. Heinemann Medical Books.
Information Folder on Practice Information Booklets. RCGP Publications.

Your Notes and Questions

Tutorial 51: Prevention and Screening

Learning Objectives

1. **Principles of prevention and screening**

2. **Opportunities for prevention**
   Smoking
   Alcohol
   Immunisation
   Home accidents

3. **Methods of Screening**
   Opportunistic versus systematic
   Diabetes
   Hypertension
   Glaucoma
   Urinary tract infection
   Breast
   Cervix
   Elderly

4. **Role of Health Education Officers**

5. **Role of Primary Health Care Team**

Trainee Self Awareness

1. How could you modify your medical records to improve preventative care?
2. What is the role of the practice nurse and health visitor in screening?
3. Does the 'item of service' payment level of a practice reflect its level of preventative care? Discuss.
4. What methods of Health Education can be used in General Practice? Name which you favour and why.

Further Reading

Practising Prevention. BMJ Publications.
Combined Reports on Prevention 18-21 (1984). Reports from General Practice. RCG publications.
Prevention and the Primary Care Team (1986). RCGP Publications.
Preventive Medicine in General Practice. J. A. M. Gray and G. H. Fowler. Oxford University Press.
Healthier Children - Thinking Prevention. Report from General Practice 22. RCGP Publications.

Your Notes and Questions

The MRCGP Examination

The number of candidates sitting the MRCGP examination each year is now approximately 1,300, and with an overall pass rate of about 70% the examination cannot be described as easy. The pass rates are better for trainees than for principals and are better for those born and educated in the UK compared with those born and educated overseas. Although the overall pass rate is higher than for some other postgraduate medical exams it is not an exam to be taken lightly. Failure is also expensive.

The examination is an "assessment of the knowledge, skills and attitudes appropriate to the general practitioner on completion of vocational training, assessing the competence of candidates to carry out unsupervised responsibility for the care of patients in general practice".

The exam syllabus covers a great breadth of knowledge and the exam itself aims to measure knowledge, skills and attitudes within the 5 areas of general practice.

1 Clinical Practice - Health and Disease
2 Clinical Practice - Human Development
3 Clinical Practice - Human Behaviour
4 Medicine and Society
5 The Practice

The syllabus is shown in detail in the RCGP publication The Future General Practitioner - Learning and Teaching, available from medical bookshops or direct from the Royal College of General Practitioners, 14 Princes Gate, Hyde Park, London SW7 1PU.

Many candidates do not appreciate the wide subject matter required and find themselves inadequately prepared to answer questions on these topics. The inadequate preparation is reflected in the results of the MRCGP exam where lower marks are scored on topics such as:

Health education
Preventive care
Practice organisation
Roles of Primary Health Care Team members
Subjects with a large ethical and/or legal basis

In the examination, (and in practice!) each area carries equal marks. The examiner is interested in the concept of whole patient care.

The object of taking the MRCGP examination is to become a member of the College, there is no other way of becoming a member.

Eligibility: usually any doctor who is eligible for the Joint Committee on Postgraduate Training for General Practice certificate (JCPTGP) is eligible to take the MRCGP examination. If there are any doubts then you should apply to the membership secretary at the Royal College.

Applications: the examination takes place twice a year, usually mid May and late October/early November. The closing date for applications is about 8 weeks before the exam. The written papers are held in several centres but the Oral is only held in Edinburgh and London.

Format: there are 5 parts to the exam each of which is of equal value. Although each part accounts for 20% of the final total, it is not necessary to pass each individual part since a good performance in one part can compensate for a poorer performance in another.

The 3 written papers are taken on one day and the 2 orals are taken on another day about 6 weeks later.

3 written papers: Multiple Choice Questions (MCQ) 2 hours
Modified Essay Questions (MEQ) 1 1/2 hours
Practice Topic Questions (PTQ) 2 hours (previously called Traditional Essay Questions).

2 orals: Oral I: Practice Profile and Log Diary 30 mins.
Oral II: Topics not covered in the first oral 30 mins.

The 3 written papers are marked first, the marks are added together and averaged out and then divided into 3 groups.

1. Candidates whose average mark is above the pass rate (usually 50%) are invited to attend the oral exam.
2. The intermediate group of candidates are also invited to attend the oral exam. They may be able to pass the exam overall if they do well in the orals despite a borderline fail on the written papers.
3. The clear fail group (approximately 20%), who do so badly in the written papers that they have no chance of passing the exam are not invited to attend the orals.

Thus approximately 80% are invited to proceed to the orals and they are then sent the Log Diary and Practice Profile for completion.

The Royal College has gone to great lengths to construct a valid and reliable exam despite the difficulties of trying to measure knowledge, skills and attitudes. For more detail on this subject refer to The MRCGP examination and its methods by Professor J H Walker. Journal of the RCGP Oct - Dec 1983.

In brief, the MRCGP exam sets out to measure knowledge, skills and attitudes in the following way and it is probably true to say that it is as difficult for the examiners as for the candidates!

Written Papers: MCQ: Knowledge is measured.
MEQ: Skills of interpretation, problem solving and attitudes in the setting of a clinical problem are measured.
PTQ: Knowledge, skills and attitudes are measured.

The Orals: these assess all 3 parameters.

The Five Areas Of General Practice

1. Clinical Practice - Health and Disease.

The candidate will be required to demonstrate a knowledge of the diagnosis, management and, where appropriate, the prevention of diseases of importance in general practice.

a. The range of the normal
b. The patterns of illness
c. The natural history of diseases
d. Prevention
e. Early diagnosis
f. Diagnostic methods and techniques
g. Management and treatment

2. Clinical practice - Human Development.

The candidate will be expected to possess a knowledge of human development and be able to demonstrate the value of this knowledge in the diagnosis and management of patients in general practice.

a. Genetics
b. Foetal development
c. Physical development in childhood, maturity and ageing
d. Intellectual development in childhood, maturity and ageing
e. Emotional development in childhood, maturity and ageing
f. The range of the normal

3. Clinical practice - Human Behaviour.

The candidates must demonstrate an understanding of human behaviour particularly as it affects the presentation and management of disease.

a. Behaviour presenting to the general practitioner
b. Behaviour in interpersonal relationships
c. Behaviour of the family
d. Behaviour in the doctor-patient relationship

4. Medicine and society

The candidate must be familiar with the common sociological and epidemiological concepts and their relevance to medical care and demonstrate a knowledge of the organisation of medical and related services in the United Kingdom and abroad.

a. Sociological aspects of health and illness
b. The uses of epidemiology
c. The organisation of medical care in the UK - comparisons with other countries
d. The relationship of medical services to other institutions of society

5. The practice

The candidate must demonstrate a knowledge of practice organisation and administration and be able to discuss critically recent developments in the evolution of general practice.

a. Practice management
b. The team
c. Financial matters
d. Premises and equipment
e. Medical records
f. Medico-legal matters
g. Research

Further Reading
MRCGP Practice Exams. J. Sandars. Pastest.

Your Notes and Questions

Appendix 1: Chronic Disease, Planning Longterm Care

Chronic disease requirea a planned approach. The following plan has been designed to include physical, physiological, and social factors and besides being a useful aide-memoire it also provides a useful revision framework for a popular question in the MRCGP examination.

1. Main roles of the General Practitioner
   - Continuity of care
     - Long term support
     - Long term medical supervision
   - Coordination of all involved in management

2. Identification
   - Screening
     - Opportunistic case finding
     - Systematic
   - Call/Recall
     - Disease Register
     - Age Sex Register
     - Computer

3. Regular Follow-ups
   - Shared Clinical Objectives (Management Protocol)
     - Information and Health Education
     - Monitor activity and progress of disease
     - Early detection and intervention to minimise preventable complications
     - Monitor progress of any unavoidable complications
     - Maintainance of general health
     - Management of acute exacerbations
   - Role of drug therapy
     - Stepped care approach
     - Compliance
     - Monitor effectiveness
     - Monitor side effects

4. Patient Self Help
   - Shared aim to live as normal as possible
   - Consider effect on:
     - Employment
     - Sexual function
     - Marriage
     - Pregnancy
     - Driving
   - Provision of aids and appliances
   - Role of Self Help Groups (see Appendix 2)

5. Role of Primary Health Care Team (see Tutorial 7)

Outline of Nursing Process

1. Assessment of Needs
2. Planning of Interventions
3. Implementation of Care Plan
4. Evaluation

6. Role of Social Services (see Tutorial 3)

7. Role of the Hospital

Out-patient: Monitoring, investigation and therapy
In-patient: Short term
Long term
Specialist Liason Nurses
Working partnership with Consultant colleagues

8. Practice Management

Efficient systems of recall
Good record system, able to demonstrate that the process of care is in action
Cooperation cards
Efficient routes of communication to all those involved in management
Audit

Appendix 2: Organizations and Self-Help Groups

Listed below are a small number of organisations and self-help groups related to specific illnesses or problems. A more extensive list can be found in the directory **'Self-Help'** compiled by Nancy Duin and published by The Bedford Square Press of the National Council for Voluntary Organisation, 26 Bedford Square, London WC1B 3HU (Approx. £2.95).

Age Concern England, Bernard Sunley House, 60 Pitcairn Road, Mitcham, Surrey CR4 3LL (Tel: 01 640 5431)

Age Concern Greater London, 54 Knatchbull Road, London SE5 9QY (Tel: 01 737 3456)

Al-Anon Family Groups, 61 Great Dover Street, London SE1 4YF (Tel: 01 403 0888)

Alcoholics Anonymous (AA), General Service Office, PO Box 1, Stonebow House Stonebow, York YO1 2NJ (Tel: 0904 644026) Greater London (Tel: 01 834 8202)

Arthritis & Rheumatism Council (ARC), 41 Eagle Street, London WC1R 4AR (Tel: 01 405 8572)

Association of Carers, First Floor, 21-23 New Road, Chatham, Kent ME4 4 (Tel: 0634 813981)

Asthma Society & Friends of the Asthma Research Council, 300 Upper Street, Islington, London N1 2XX (Tel: 01 226 2260)

British Agencies for Adoption & Fostering (BAAF), 11 Southwark Street,London SE1 1RQ (Tel: 01 407 8800)

British Diabetic Association, 10 Queen Anne Street, London W1M 0BD (Tel: 01 323 1531)

British Epilepsy Association, Crowthorne House, Bigshotte, New Wokingham Road, Wokingham, Berkshire RG11 3AY (Tel: 0344 773122)

British Heart Foundation, 102 Gloucester Place, London W1H 4DH (Tel: 01 935 0185)

Cot Death Research & Support Associations, Foundation for the Study of Infant Death, 15 Belgrave Street, London SW1X 8PS (Tel: 01 235 1721)

Cruse: National Organisation for the Widowed and their Children, Cruse House, 126 Sheen Road, Richmond, Surrey TW9 1UR (Tel: 01 940 4818/9047)

Medical Commission on Accident Prevention, 35-43 Lincoln's Inn Fields, London WC2A 3PN (Tel: 01 242 3176)

MIND (National Association for Mental Health), 22 Harley Street, London W1N 2ED (Tel: 01 637 0741)

Miscarriage Association, 18 Stoneybrook Close, West Bretton, Wakefield,West Yorkshire WF4 4TP (Tel: 0924 85515)

Organisations and Self-Help Groups

National Eczema Society, Tavistock House North, Tavistock Square, LondonWC1H 9SR (Tel: 01 388 4097)

National Society for Prevention of Cruelty to Children (NSPCC), 67 Saffron Hill, London EC1N 8RS (Tel: 01 242 1626)

Psoriasis Association, 7 Milton Street, Northampton NN2 7JG (Tel: 0604 711129)

Samaritans, 17 Uxbridge Road, Slough, Berkshire SL1 1SN (Tel: 0753 32713/4)

Terrence Higgins Trust, BM AIDS, London WC1N 3XX (Tel: 01 833 2971)

Appendix 3: Further Reading and Reference Books

The books and booklets listed below are referred to in relevant tutorials and are recommended by the authors as a valuable foundation for any General Practice Library.

Bain J. et al. **Colour Atlas of Mouth, Throat and Ear Disorders in Children.** MTP Press.

Balint E. & Norrell J. S. **Six Minutes for the Patient: Interactions in General Practice Consultation.** Tavistock Publications.

Balint M. **The Doctor, His Patient and the Illness.** Pitman.

Balint M. Hunt J. Joyce D. Marinker M. L. & Woodcock J. **Treatment or Diagnosis.** Tavistock Publications.

Banks A. & Waller T.A.N. **Drug Addiction and Polydrug Abuse.** Institute for the Study of Drug Dependency, 1-4 Hatton Place, London EC1N 8ND

Berne E. **Games People Play.** Penguin.

BMJ Publications:
ABC of AIDS.
ABC of Alcohol.
ABC of Asthma.
ABC of Diabetes.
ABC of ENT.
ABC of Healthy Travel.
ABC of Hypertension.
ABC of 1-7.
ABC of Ophthalmology.
ABC of Practical Procedures.
ABC of Sexually Transmitted Diseases.
Blood Pressure Measurement.
Employing Staff.
Medicine in Old Age.
Organising a Practice.
Practising Prevention.
The Handbook of Medical Ethics.

Brooks D. & Dunbar E. M. **Infectious Diseases in General Practice.** MTP Press.

Brooks D. & Mallick N. **Renal Medicine and Urology.** Library of General Practice, Volume 4. Churchill Livingstone.

Byrne P. S. & Long B. E. L. **Doctors Talking to Patients.** HMSO, London.

Byrne A. & Padfield C. **Social Services.** Made Simple Books. Heinemann.

Clark T. & Rees J. **Practical Management of Asthma.** Dunitz.

Coni N. Davison W. & Webster S. **Lecture Notes on Geriatrics.** Blackwell Scientific Publications.

Coope J. **The Menopause.** BMA Family Doctor Publications.

Cormack J. Marinker M. & Morrell D. **Practice, A Handbook of Primary Medical Care.** Kluwer Medical.

DHSS. **Drug Tariff.**
Handbook of Contraceptive Practice.
Immunisation against Infectious Diseases.
Medical Evidence for Social Security Purposes.

Ellis N. **Employing Staff.** BMJ Publications.

Freeling P. & Harris C. M. **The Doctor-Patient Relationship.** Churchill Livingstone.

Fry J. **Common Diseases, their Nature, Incidence and Care.** MTP Press.

Fry J. **Present State and Future Needs in General Practice.** For RCGP, MTP Press.

Fuller & Toon **Medical Practice in a Multicultural Society.** Heinemann Medical Books.

Gee D. **Lecture Notes on Forensic Medicine.** Blackwell Scientific Publications.

Gelder M. et al. **Oxford Textbook of Psychiatry.** Oxford University Press.

General Medical Council. **Professional Conduct and Disipline: fitness to practice.**

Gray J. A. M. & Fowler G. H. **Preventive Medicine in General Practice.** Oxford University Press.

Hart J. T. & Stilwell B. **Prevention of Coronary Heart Disease and Stroke.** Faber & Faber.

Howie J. **Research and General Practice.** Croom Helm.

Illingworth R. S. **Basic Developmental Screening: 0-4 years.** Blackwell Scientific Publications.

Illingworth R. S. **The Normal Child.** Churchill Livingstone.

Insley J. & Wood B. **A Paediatric Vade-mecum.** Lloyd-Luke.

Jayson M. I. V. & Million R. **Locomotor Disability in General Practice.** Oxford University Press.

Jones R. V. H. et al. **Running a Practice.** Croom Helm.

Kaye P. **Notes for the DRCOG.** Churchill Livingstone.

Lancaster-Smith M. J. & Chapman C. **Gastroenterology.** MTP Press.

Levene G. M. & Calnan C. D. **A Colour Atlas of Dermatology.** Wolfe Medical.

McKie R. **Clinical Dermatology - an Illustrated Textbook.** Oxford University Press.

McPherson A. & Anderson A. **Women's Problems in General Practice.** Oxford University Press.

Moulds A. J. Martin P. B. & Bouchier Hayes T. A. **Emergencies in General Practice.** MTP Press.

Munro E. Manthei R. J. & Small J. J. **Counselling: a Skills Approach.** Methuen.

Neighbour R. **The Inner Consultation.** MTP Press.

Oxford GP Group. **A Guide to General Practice.** Blackwell Scientific Publications.

Pendleton D. **The Consultation: An Approach to Learning & Teaching.** Oxford University Press.

Pollak M. & Fry J. **Commonsense Paediatrics.** MTP Press.

Potts M. & Diggory P. **Contraceptive Practice.** Cambridge University Press.

Preece J. **The Use of Computers in General Practice.** Churchill Livingstone.

Pritchard P. M. M. **Practice Management.** Oxford University Press.

RCGP Publications:

Alcohol: A Balanced View. 1986. Reports from General Practice 24.
An Atlas of Bedside Microscopy. Occasional Paper 32.
Booking for Maternity Care, a Comparison of Two Systems. Occasional Paper 31.
Combined Reports on Prevention 18-21. Reports from General Practice.
Healthier Children: Thinking Prevention. Reports from General Practice 22.
In Pursuit of Quality.
Information Folder on Age/Sex Registers.
Information Folder on Appointment Systems.
Information Folder on Asthma.
Information Folder on Cervical Cytology.
Information Folder on Diabetes.
Information Folder on Epilepsy.
Information Folder on Medical Records.
Information Folder on Parkinson's Disease.
Information Folder on Practice Information Booklet.
Inner Cities. Occasional Paper 19.
Management in Practice (video package).
Medical Audit in General Practice. Occasional Paper 20.
Patient Participation in General Practice. Occasional Paper 17.
Present State and Future Needs in General Practice.
Preventive Care of the Elderly. Occasional Paper 35.
Prevention and the Primary Care Team.
Quality in General Practice. Policy Statement 2.
Social Class and Health Status. Inequality or Difference. Occasional Paper 25.
The Presentation of Depression: Current Approaches. Occasional Paper 36.
The Work of Counsellors in General Practice. Occasional Paper 37.

Trainee Projects. Occasional Paper 29.
What sort of doctor? Reports from General Practice 23.

Sandars J. **MRCGP Practice Exams.** PasTest.

Sneddon I. & Church R. **Practical Dermatology.** Edward Arnold.

Spilling R. **Terminal Care.** Oxford University Press.

Stott N. C. H. & Davis R. H. **The Exceptional Potential in Each Primary Care Consultation.** Journal of the RCGP 29:201-5. (1979)

Tudor Hart J. **Hypertension.** Churchill Livingstone.

Worden W. **Grief Therapy.** Tavistock Publications.

Miscellaneous:

British National Formulary (BNF)

Medical Aspects of Fitness to Drive. Medical Commission on Accident Prevention, 50 Old Brompton Road, London SW7 3EA.

Pulse 'Blue Book'. Published yearly by Pulse Magazine.

Statement of Fees and Allowances (SFA) 'The Red Book'. The Family Practioner Committee (FPC).

Notes

Notes